Running to Lose Weight Using Weight Training and Cardio

How to Lose Weight Using Running and Weights

Table of Contents

Introduction

Chapter 1: The Benefits of Losing Weight via Running

Chapter 2: Lose Weight By Running
    Section 1: Spirit
    Section 2: Habit Forming
    Section 3: Choosing a Pace

Chapter 3: Healthy Eating Habits
    Section 1: Eating Before Your Workout
    Section 2: Eating After You Work Out
    Section 3: Differentiated Eating Habits

Chapter 4: Losing Weight with Weight Training

Chapter 5: How to Lose Weight Generally
    Tip 1: Move
    Tip 2: Track Your Fitness
    Tip 3: Make your Weight Loss a Contest
    Tip 4: Find Small Breaks
    Tip 5: Cook at Home
    Tip 6: Walk Rather Than Drive

Conclusion

Introduction

Hello, dear reader, and thank you for picking up the ebook "Running to Lose Weight Using Weight Training and Cardio." This book is a short, but comprehensive, beginner's guide to understanding the basics of losing weight through daily exercise (primarily running, as the title suggests) with weight training thrown in to help balance your exercise routine.

The point of this book, and you reading through its pages, is to guide you through the basics and early stages of creating and sticking to a healthy cardio-based exercise routine to help you shed a few pounds.

It should be noted that, while there are tons of different kinds of exercise routines and workouts out there, this book focuses on running, cardio, and weight lifting with the purpose of weight lose. This book will not delve into the complex world of muscle building and extensive dieting (although the latter will come into play throughout these pages).

I hope you find this beginner's guide helpful and enjoyable to read.

Chapter 1: The Benefits of Losing Weight via Running

First thing's first: What are the benefits you can reap by running on a daily basis? Well, as the title suggests, one of the primary reasons to run is to lose weight. Like most exercises, running won't give you instantaneous results (you're not going to lose ten pounds in a week), but once you make running a part of your everyday routine, you'll shed weight with relatively little effort.

Not only will you lose weight, you'll keep that weight off if you continue to run. Running daily will keep your body in good shape and keep your weight down.

Unlike the weight lose, one thing you will notice right away is that you'll feel all around better. You'll feel healthier and will have more energy throughout the day. That's one of the best parts about running and other exercises:

You won't have that caffeine crash a few hours later (unlike coffee).

With more energy comes a generally healthier sleeping schedule. You may not feel a crash right after lunch due to running, but you will begin to feel tired earlier in the evening (for you night owls, running at night may be a better option). When you feel more tired in the evening, you'll find it easier to fall asleep, which can lead to overall better sleep throughout the night.

Really, the benefits of running come in all shapes and sizes. From keeping your body healthy, to forming a healthier sleeping habit. Some would go as far as to say running works in a similar fashion to meditating (which I am inclined to agree with) as running gives you that much needed "me time" in the day.

While all of these benefits are fantastic ways to improve your quality of life in the long run, it's not an easy path to get to the point where these benefits are noticeable. There's a long trek ahead of you, but this book is here to help guide you through those tough times.

Chapter 2: Lose Weight By Running

Running is one of the best (and easiest) ways to lose weight and keep your weight down through day to day practices. Relative to a lot of other exercises and workouts, running can be less intensive, but still provide great results in a relatively short amount of time. You won't drop down to five percent body fat overnight, however. Running does take persistence, determination, and several days of hating the activity before you fully start to experience the benefits the exercise has to offer.

In this chapter, we will discuss the three basic guidelines to help you get the most out of your running routine. These guidelines cover things like how to stay positive and willing to run even when it feels awful, how to form a habit to help your running routine become a part of your everyday, how to set a pace for your running to best maximize your efforts, and how to make the most of your progress toward weight lose with simple eating habits.

While the four sections in this chapter all work to a degree individually, they should be combined into your daily routine to really make the most of your time spent exercising.

Section 1: Spirit

One of the hardest parts of, well, anything is simply getting up and starting it. Especially when it comes to exercising and running, a wall can stand in your way to get out of bed and start your day with a run.

If you want to lose any amount of weight through running, you will have to push past any excuses to *not* run. For example, running in the morning is a great way to start any day and will do a heck of a lot more to wake you up than any size cup of coffee. The only challenge is physically getting up, getting prepared, and walking out that door without any help from coffee. This is where determination comes in. You have to want to go running and lose weight. The more you consider running (or any exercise) a chore, the harder it will be to start it, and the easier it will be to procrastinate.

I can tell you now, for any of you readers who are beginning to run routinely for the first time: There will be plenty of days (especially at the beginning) that you won't want to run. In those early days, you'll find plenty of excuses not to run and to stay in bed, or to finish watching one more episode of a show.

Simply put, in those early days of running, you won't want to run when it comes time to start your exercise. This isn't a bad thing, it's how humans are designed. What is important, however, is that you learn how to push past these feelings of "Oh, I'll just do it later." This is easier than it sounds. All it takes is for you to form a habit.

Section 2: Habit Forming

Habits are relatively difficult to form, and incredibly easy to break (unless they're bad habits, that is). For something like running every morning (or every night), the habit forming process is long and probably one of the most frustrating things you will ever go through.

On average, it takes an individual roughly twenty one days of doing something to form a habit. What that means is, for three weeks of your life, you will have to wake up and get up to run, despite your body telling you that it doesn't want to. These first three weeks are the hardest part of any habit, and will be the worst three weeks of running in your life.

However, once those three weeks are up and you ran every morning for your set amount of time or distance, it only gets easier. Once the habit is formed, you will find your body automatically pumping itself up each morning to go on a run. No longer will you feel sluggish to waking up, you'll be up and ready to go.

But, you may be wondering, how can I force myself up when even my body doesn't want to get up and go? There's a simple solution to this that can be the difference between making and breaking your running habit: Assign the task of waking you up to something else.

No, I don't mean hire one of your friends to come wake you up each and every morning to start your run. What I do mean is, simply, set an alarm to get you going in the morning. If you're like a large percent of people, you'll find it all too easy to turn over, hit snooze and fall right back asleep.

This is where yet another habit comes in: Waking up with your alarm. Like running or other exercise, you need to train your body to wake up at a specific time. If your alarm goes off, and your first instinct is to turn it off and return to your warm blankets, you will not find waking up easy. If, however, you train yourself to get up on the first alarm, you'll have a much easier time.

How can you become better at setting your wake up schedule? For starters, force yourself to wake up. That's the first major step. If you can force your legs over the side of your bed as soon as that alarm goes off, you're in good shape. If that continues to be a problem, you may want to set your alarm clock or cell phone way on the other side of the room so you're forced to stand up and walk to it to turn it off.

There are a ton of fun little alarm clocks that make you do some activity to turn them off (from shooting a target with a laser gun, to physically chasing a small car around your room). While those are fun novelties, you don't want your body to rely on that kind of stimulus to wake up. The goal here is to form the habit of waking up right as your alarm goes off regardless of how close it is or how easily you can turn it off.

Say that you are still finding it difficult to wake up even after trying several alarm tricks. You just can't find the motivation to get up and run. Don't sweat it, that's very understandable. If you do find yourself still struggling (and remember, you will struggle for the first three weeks or so), then you can try sharing the responsibility with a friend or family member.

While waking up to fulfill a promise to yourself can be difficult, you may find it easier to find a running body to help share the responsibility. Rather than waking up for your own needs, you'll have to wake up for someone else. In this instance, you and your friend have to wake up at the same time, which provides two major benefits to forming a habit:

1) A partner to help carry the responsibility - - Now, if you do sleep in by mistake (forgot to set your alarm, didn't charge your phone, hit snooze and fell back asleep, whatever reason), you'll have your partner to act as a net. The chance of both of you sleeping in is far less than one of you.

2) You no longer have just a responsibility to yourself -- Rather than forming a running habit for your own health, you now have

someone else who relies on you waking up and running to help them. If you need to wake up to help someone else, chances are you will find yourself waking up easier.

In short, forming a habit is the first essential part to running to lose weight. While the proper attitude and spirit helps quite a bit, it is almost impossible to have that go-getter attitude right out of the gate. Forming a habit will, simply, make your entire running experience easier and an essential part of your everyday life. Not to mention, if you do it long enough, your body will crave that daily run.

Once the waking up portion is beginning to slide into place and you find yourself forcing yourself to run every day, there will be other reasons not to run. For example, there will be days during those first three weeks where you'll wake up with your legs aching too much to move -- or so you think.

They will hurt, don't get me wrong, but they will only hurt until you start to run again. Once you get up, get out, and start running, you'll notice your legs will feel better. And, as you do this day after day, that hurt will come back less and less.

There is one bit of advice that has helped me form a habit and stick to it: Set a schedule (or set a time everyday or however many times a week), keep it consistent, and when it's time to do something, get up and do it with no hesitation. If you set an alarm for every morning at six, as soon as that alarm goes off, get up and go. Don't think about it because that will only make starting more difficult.

Section 3: Choosing a Pace

It's important for any part of your habit forming and post habit forming time to set a pace that works for you. If you work too hard in the early days of your running routine, you will tire yourself out too quickly and not reap the benefits of running long term. If, on the other hand, you don't work out hard enough, you will find it to be easier, but your body won't adjust to the heart-pumping exercise you need to lose weight.

Like any and all workouts, the first rule is one that everyone may remember from middle school fitness class: Warm up and cool down before and after every workout.

These steps are important for several reasons:

1) Warming up will allow your muscles to stretch and loosen up. If you remember anything from middle or high school, it's that warmed up muscles have a lower chance of cramping or aching during a workout.
2) Warming your body up helps start a workout with an already increased heart rate. This will make it easier to get to a nice elevated heart rate throughout your running.
3) A cool down will help your heart rate decrease at a slower rate. Rather than going from a running heart rate to a full stop (a resting heart rate), which can cause chest pains and momentary

breathing problems, your body will lower its heart rate over a longer time. This makes the transition from workout mode to resting mode smoother.

4) Cooling your body down after a workout will help prevent future aches and pains.

While warming up and cooling down help set the pace of your pre and post workout respectively, there's one major issue that still needs to be addressed: How do you choose how fast, far, and long to run?

Well, those are really up to you. Obviously, the longer and further you run, the more you'll get out of your work out. That said, there is a few things you should consider before just running for hours into the horizon.

1) It's not about finishing up your run in a short a time as possible. It's really the opposite. If you want to reap the most benefits of your run, you want a mildly paced, longer run to help you build up stamina and lose weight over time.

2) A fast pace is not always a good thing. You never want to full on sprint during your run (unless you're practicing for a short distance run like the one hundred meter sprint). That will only increase your heart rate too quickly and leave you out of breath.

3) Alternate between running and walking (especially for the first several weeks). You'll find yourself getting way too tired if you try to run constantly. Walk for a few minutes, then run for a few minutes. This will help keep your heart rate up and increase your exercise time drastically.

4) Never just stop moving. As long as you feel alright and not light headed or dizzy, keep moving (either running, walking, or jogging in place). If you stop moving to sit down, you'll heart rate will begin to decrease almost instantly and you'll find it difficult to stand up and continue.

This may seem like a good chunk of information to remember, but once you begin to remind yourself every day of these practices, they will become second nature.

Listening to music (or audiobooks) is also a great way to help keep your pace up. If you have a workout playlist full of fast electronica music, keep in mind that each song is roughly on average three and a half minutes long (which makes a great time for switching from running to walking).

There are also tons of apps that help you set your pace. If you browse the iPhone App store, Google Play, or even the Amazon App Marketplace, you'll find tons of different themed apps that revolve around keeping you moving while out and about. These range from a simple time that beeps when you switch from running to walking and vice versa, to a full on narrative about zombies infecting your town (be careful not to walk too slowly, though, or else the zombies can get you).

If you're finding running to be a bit boring, find a playlist, a book, or a fun app to help keep you motivated as you lose weight and get healthier.

Chapter 3: Healthy Eating Habits

A common mistake while running is having the wrong kind of eating habits. There are several aspects to eating that can affect either your workout itself, or the results from your workout.

Depending on your workout of choice, whether it be running, weight lifting, swimming, etc., and your ultimate end goal to working out, your eating habits will vary.

It should go without saying, but always stay hydrated during your run. Keeping water with you will help prevent dehydration.

Section 1: Eating Before Your Workout

One strongly misunderstood factor of a workout is eating before hand. There are tons of misconceptions about eating prior to a workout regardless of intensity.

Many people assume that you don't want to eat any food prior to your workout (I mean, why would you eat food when you're trying to lose weight, right?). The simple facts are, you need to eat something before working out to give your body the proper energy to actually work out. Say you want to work out first thing in the morning, but don't eat anything before you do so. You're going to feel weak either during or shortly after your run.

You want to eat before hand. Simple as that. But how much you eat is a different animal altogether. You want to eat a small amount of food to get sugar to your blood. Fruits work well for this reason because of that burst of energy you'll get from their natural sugars.

You do not, however, want to have a full meal right before you go out. Eating too much can cause you to feel sick when you're out and about. Keep it small, keep it light, and be sure to eat about twenty minutes before you actually start (you want to give that food time to settle).

Another benefit to eating before hand is the jump start the food will give your metabolism. If you don't eat, your metabolism won't kick on and you won't lost as much weight.

In short, there is no positive benefit to not eating something small before going on a run. Grab a banana on the way out the door. That's all it takes.

Section 2: Eating After You Work Out

After your run is the time to grab a nice hearty breakfast (or supper, or lunch). At this point, your metabolism will be turned to its highest and you'll probably be craving something to refill your energy. You won't be sleepy tired anymore, so that morning cup of joe isn't necessary at this point (but it is always enjoyable and healthy if you drink it black).

Spend some time to prepare a nice meal with natural sugars, protein, and carbs to allow your body to refuel and make the most of the foods you eat. It's best if you fit in your meal about half an hour after your workout to get the most of the foods and their nutrients.

Section 3: Differentiated Eating Habits

As I mentioned earlier, you're going to have different eating habits based on what your end goals are. For example, if you want to run to lose weight and feel healthier, you're going to eat lighter foods such as fruits and vegetables.

If, however, your goal is to add muscle to your body, then you're going to want to include more protein to add to those muscles.

Running, on its own, doesn't build a lot of muscle because you're not pushing any particular muscle past its limits. It will, however, work to tone the muscles you already have to make them more efficient. Eating a lot of protein if you're only running will only place protein in your body with nowhere to go (unlike heavy weight lifting, during which the muscles are pushed past their limits and allowed to be built up). That's why it's essential to eat fruits, vegetables, and small amounts of carb based foods (pastas are always a good choice). The fruits offer sugars to keep you going, the vegetables satisfy your hunger without an excess of calories, and the carbs will help keep you running longer (but remember, only in small amounts).

Your daily eating habits also play a big role with your weight loss. You could run ten miles every day, but if you go home and eat only sugary foods, candies, and high fat products, you won't lose any weight (albeit, it would take several cakes to balance a daily run of ten miles).

The most influential thing you can do regarding your eating habits is pay attention to portions. Sure, you can go to the local Olive Garden and get a plate of spaghetti after a run, but that plate of spaghetti is, in reality, at least three servings of pasta (that's right, a full day's amount). People always want to eat more than they should because we're inclined to believe a meal from a restaurant is really that, a meal, when really it can have enough calories for two, three, four, even five meals.

Mentioning calories, keep track. You don't need to write down the exact amount of calories you eat with every meal, but know your daily limit (I use the Super Tracker at www.Supertracker.usda.gov to find my daily allowance) and eat accordingly. If you want to lose weight then eat less than your daily amount, if you want to gain weight then eat more, and if you want to stay the same then eat roughly your daily allotment.

Chapter 4: Losing Weight with Weight Training

I've brought up weightlifting and weight training too many times in previous chapters to not talk about its benefits.

The largest difference between running and weight training lies within the use of muscles with either exercise. While running (and other cardio exercises) slim you down and tone muscles, weight training helps preserve those muscles while dropping fat.

If you want to lose weight in general (muscle and fat), run.

If you want to lose fat, but maintain muscle, weight train.

Shockingly, weight training works similar to running, in that you don't want to over exert yourself too quickly. Rather, you want to abide by the classic advice: Lower weight with more reps. When you do a lower weight, you don't stress your muscles, but rather you tone them and melt away fat. This is similar to long range running in that it's a longer workout with relatively less stress.

If, however, you did want to bulk up, you would do the opposite: More weight with fewer reps. The heavier weight will push your muscles to their limit allowing for protein to build upon them. This is the workout for which you would want to eat more protein. But, as muscle weighs more than fat, you may find yourself gaining muscle mass.

Now that you know the basics of weight training, and the difference between the types, the question pops up again: How does one lose weight lifting weights?

To lose weight lifting weights, you abide by the same basic rules of running. You want to eat a small amount of food before you workout, you want to warm up and cool down, and you want to do an extended, light intensity workout to help maintain a moderately high heart rate for a longer period of time.

Also, like running, lifting weights can take time to make into a habit. You will have to struggle for a few weeks before making weight training into a part of your every day or week.

Chapter 5: How to Lose Weight Generally

Now that we've covered the basics of running and weight training, we can discuss other ways to implement weight loss into your everyday life. I know what you are thinking: "I'm already running every morning, what else do you want me to do?"

Don't worry, I'm not going to tell you to strap weights to your ankles or to skip instead of walk (although both would help you lose more weight). These are simple tricks to help you get the most of your day to day life.

Tip 1: Move

For starters, simply move more. When you're cleaning your house, why not put on music and dance? Those extra hip swings and dance moves will add up to help you lose calories while doing daily chores. Sure, you may feel a bit silly doing it, but it's your house, so who cares? Plus if anyone makes fun of you, it's their loss because you're losing weight and having a blast doing so!

Tip 2: Track Your Fitness

The second tip is preference, but many many people like to have a fitness tracking device to help them keep track of daily steps and workout time. Devices like Fitbit, Under Armour, Garmin, Smartwatches, and even Google and Apple have fitness trackers. Some you can wear on your wrist or bra strap, others use your phone to track your daily fitness. For many, it helps to have a visual reminder of how well they're doing on a day to day basis.

The ability to set up challenges with friends and have an hourly reminder to get up and move help a lot when trying to lose weight.

Tip 3: Make your Weight Loss a Contest

Like the Fitbit allows, making a competition out of working out or losing weight makes it not only more fun, but offers a bit more incentive for keeping the habit strong. Whether it's a friendly competition between friends, or an office-wide contest for bragging rights (or more tangible prizes), making weight loss into a contest can be a great way to push yourself to do more.

Tip 4: Find Small Breaks

If you're not doing anything important, why not take a step outside and walk around the block. Even something as simple as a five minute stroll can add up if you do it everyday.

Are you a fan of video games? While the game takes a few moments to load, why not get on the ground and do five pushups? If you sit in front of the couch for hours at a time, you may know how many loading screens can come up. If you do five pushups per loading screen, and you encounter maybe ten every hour, that's fifty pushups and hour, which will definitely help you lose weight faster.

Tip 5: Cook at Home

I know how easy it is to stop at McDonald's on the way home from work after a stressful day, but each product on their menu is chalk full of calories and sugars.

If you spend half an hour preparing food, not only will you work up an appetite, you'll know exactly what ingredients are going into your mouth and can adjust them if they seem too fatty.

A slow cooker or crock pot can do wonders for those with busy schedules, too. You spend maybe twenty minutes prepping the food (often times, recipes require you just throw ingredients into the crock pot), and in five to ten hours you will have a delicious meal waiting for you.

"Five to ten hours?" You may shout in outrage. "I would have starved to death by then!"

I can see where you are coming from, but consider this: if you prepare the food the night before, right before you go to bed, you can wake up with a steaming, fresh meal waiting for you the next morning. No need to cook anything right when you get back from your morning run, it'll be ready for you as you walk through the door (the same works with long days at the office).

Tip 6: Walk Rather Than Drive

If you live a mile away from the grocery store (or your favorite bar) why not spend twenty or so minutes to walk rather than drive. Now, of course there will be times when you need to pick up several bags of groceries, so walking is out of the question. That's fine. But if you forgot the hot sauce for taco night, there's no harm in spending some extra time to walk to the store to grab some.

There's more benefits to this, too. If you walk to the bar, there's no risk of you driving home after your fifth beer and third shot. It'll keep you safer because you'll have to walk back. Walking will also limit your night -- you don't want to walk home at three in the morning, so you'll maybe head back at eleven instead. This helps keep your sleeping habits in check and can help save you from making poor decisions (plus, you'll walk off all those shots of tequila).

Conclusion

Thank you for picking up and reading "Running to Lose Weight Using Weight Training and Cardio." I hope you found some of these tips helpful to your weight loss goals.

And, yes, losing weight is hard, but it gets easier over time and soon you'll be looking and feeling better than you ever thought possible.

Good luck!

www.ingramcontent.com/pod-product-compliance
Lightning Source LLC
Chambersburg PA
CBHW071316280526
45788CB00004B/1914